Taboo Cancer Cures

Six Easy Things You Can Do to Avoid Getting Cancer

By Paul Magnolia

Legal Notice:

This eBook is copyright protected. This is only for personal use. You cannot amend, distribute, sell, use, quote or paraphrase any part or the content within this eBook without the consent of the author or copyright owner. Legal action will be pursued if this is breached.

Disclaimer Notice:

Please note the information contained within this document is for educational purposes only.

Every attempt has been made to provide accurate, up to date and reliable complete information no warranties of any kind are expressed or implied. Readers acknowledge that the author is not engaging in rendering legal, financial or professional advice.

By reading any document, the reader agrees that under no circumstances are we responsible for any losses, direct or indirect, which are incurred as a result of use of the information contained within this document, including – but not limited to errors, omissions, or inaccuracies.

Table of Contents

Introduction……………………………………………………………pg. 5

The Anti-Cancer Diet……………………………………………….pg. 8

Anti-Cancer Vitamins……………………………………………….pg. 14

Anti-Cancer Exercise………………………………………………pg. 18

Anti-Cancer Yoga…………………………………………………..pg. 23

Anti-Cancer Products……………………………………………..pg. 28

Anti-Cancer Habits……………………………………………..pg. 33

Conclusion……………………………………………………..pg. 38

Introduction

Cancer is a disease that can affect anybody. It strikes seemingly without warning, and it can impact people of all ages. There are many things that can contribute to cancer, including hereditary factors and environmental factors. Sometimes, people who do everything they can to live healthy lives still end up with a diagnosis of cancer.

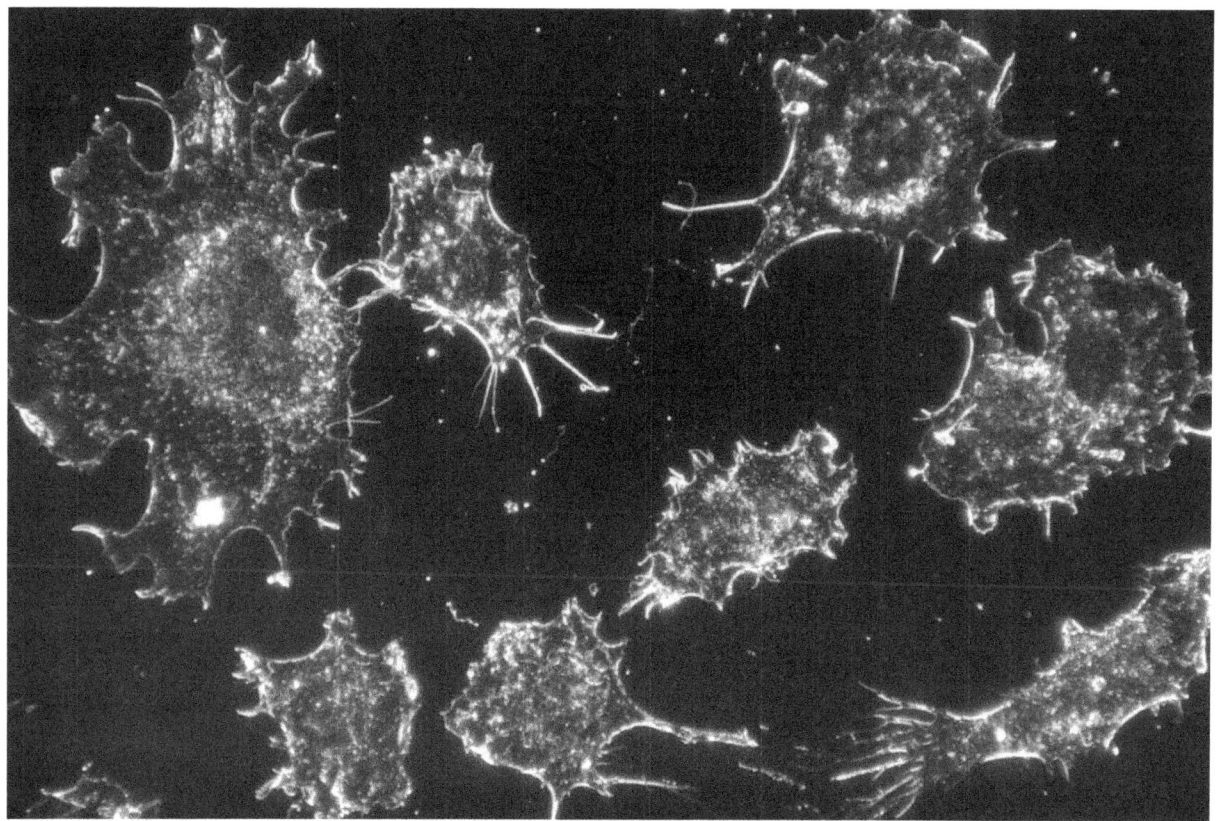

In some cases, getting cancer may be beyond our control. However, there are things that we can do to reduce our risk of getting it.

What You Will Learn in This Book

Researchers work every day to find a cure for cancer, but as the saying goes, an ounce of prevention is worth a pound of cure. That's why I tell my patients about simple things they can do to minimize the chances that they will get cancer – and now I want to share those things with you, too.

The information in this book breaks down into six categories – six areas where you can make smart choices that will give your body what it needs to resist cancer and stay healthy. Here's what I'll cover:

- Diet. Many types of cancer can be linked to the unhealthy food we eat. I'll tell you about the foods that are most likely to cause cancer, as well as those that can help to prevent it.
- Vitamins. Not all supplements are helpful, but there are some micronutrients and herbs that play a big role in helping to ward off cancer.
- Exercise. Certain kinds of cancer are directly linked to your percentage of body fat, and exercise is the best way to reduce your body fat and protect yourself.
- Yoga. I am giving Yoga its own category because it plays an important role in terms of detoxifying and strengthening your body.
- Products. Many of the products we use on a daily basis, including cleaning products and cosmetics, contain harsh chemicals and known carcinogens. I'll tell you which ingredients to avoid and suggest healthy alternatives.

- Habits. Do you have healthy habits? Things like what type of water you drink and how much you sleep can have a direct impact on your risk of getting cancer.

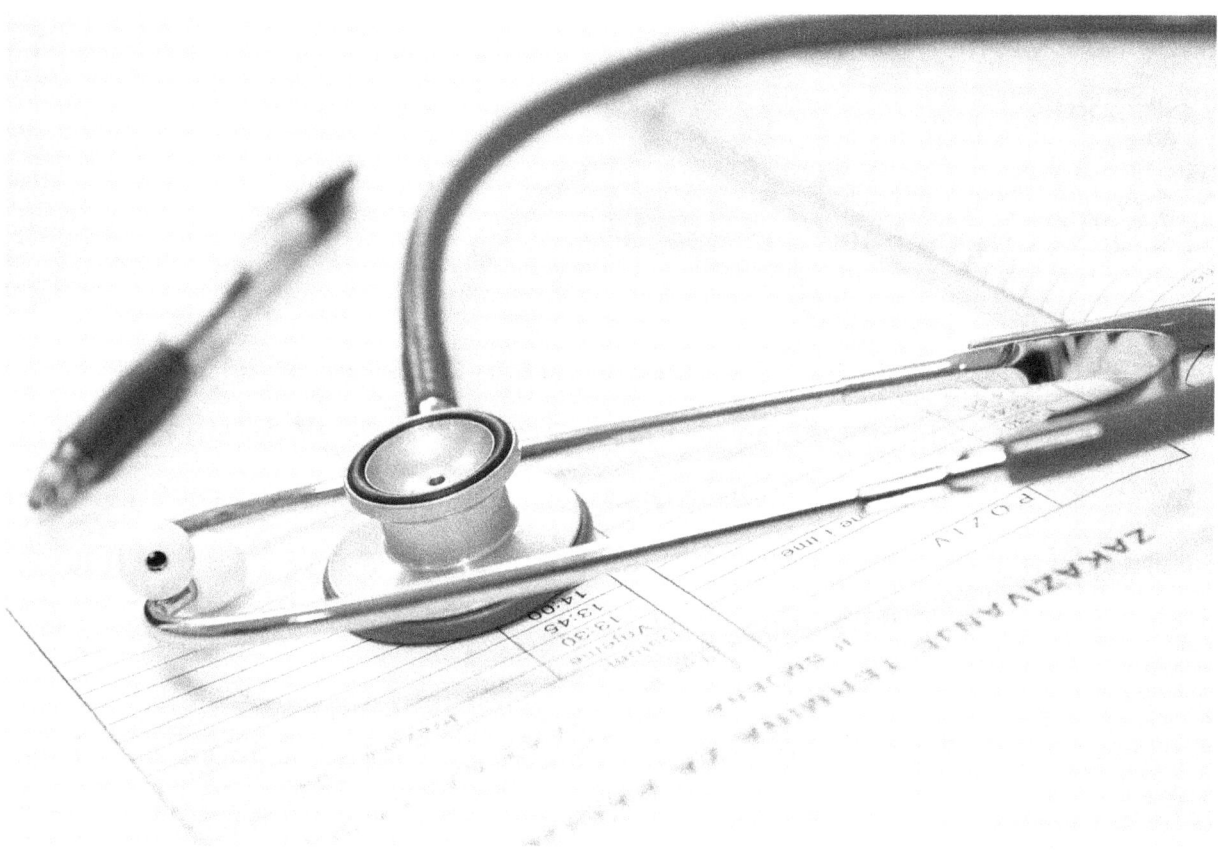

By the time you are finished with this book, you will have the same valuable information I give to my patients – the information that can help you make healthy changes that will greatly reduce your risk of getting cancer.

Do you want to live a long and healthy life? This book can help you do that.

Let's get started.

The Anti-Cancer Diet

The first topic I want to cover is one that gets quite a bit of attention. As the saying goes, "You are what you eat." On some level I think we all know that to be true, yet many of us eat foods that are detrimental to our health and wellbeing.

The Link between Food and Health

Let's start by talking about why diet and health are so intertwined. The simplest analogy I can use is one that many people will understand. If you have a car that uses gasoline and you give it diesel fuel, it will not run properly. The same is true if you try to use gasoline in a vehicle that has a diesel engine. Using the right fuel matters.

Food is fuel. Your body uses food to function. For example, there are three macronutrients: carbohydrates, proteins, and fats. Your body uses carbohydrates as its first source of energy. Proteins are the building blocks of muscle and perform other important functions in the body. Fats help to lubricate your joints and digestive system. You need all three to be healthy.

The same is true of micronutrients, which you may know by their more common names, vitamins and minerals. Let's look at just one example. Vitamin C is an antioxidant, which means that it protects your cells against a type of damage known as oxidative stress. It also boosts the immune system, supports healthy bones and teeth, and aids in tissue repair. Every other essential vitamin and mineral plays multiple roles in the body, helping to keep you healthy and strong.

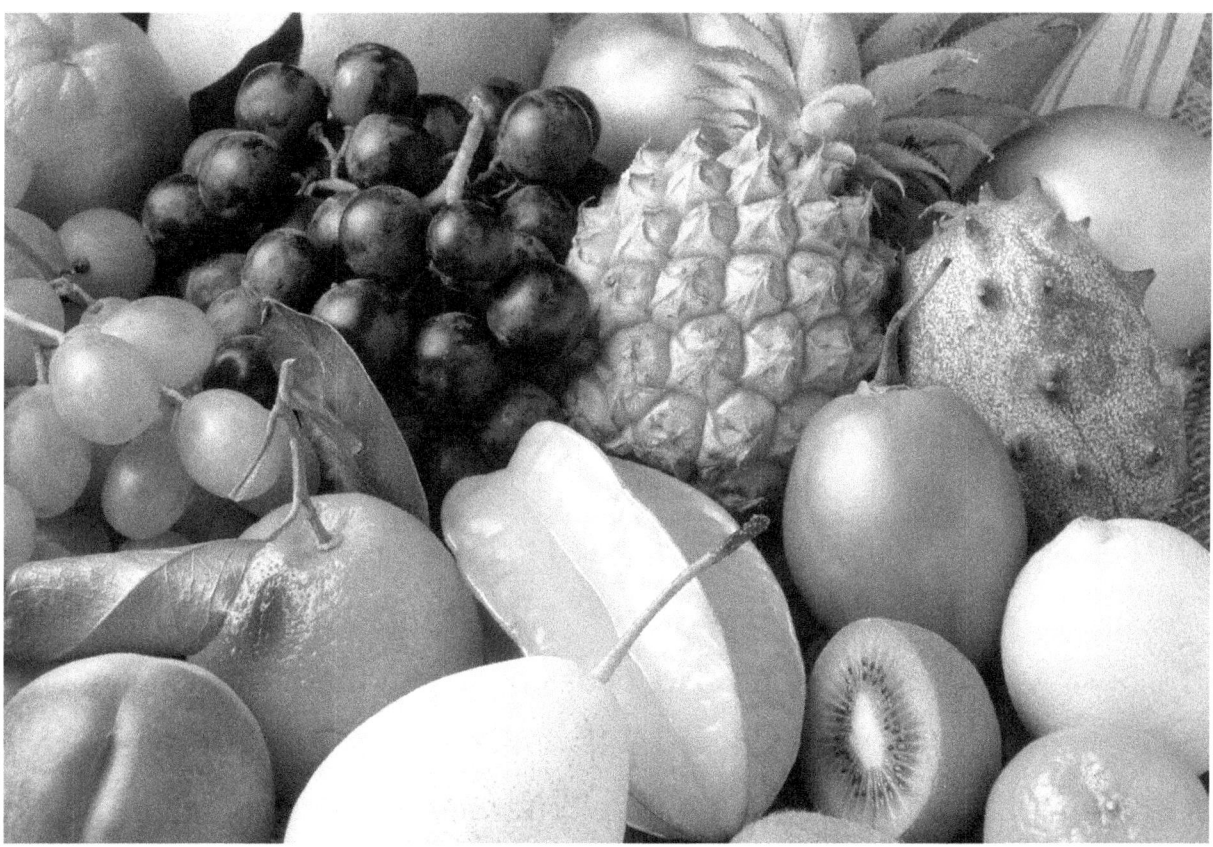

Why You Should Eat Organic

One of the most important things you can do to prevent cancer is to eat organic fruits and vegetables. Factory farmed produce is often grown with the use of pesticides that contain known carcinogenic substances. Organic produce is strictly regulated and is much safer to eat than non-organic produce.

The same goes for organic animal protein and products. Often, large food manufacturers feed livestock with unhealthy food such as corn, which is high in inflammatory Omega-6 essential fatty acid. They also pump the animals full of antibiotics and growth hormones, all of which can play a role in causing cancer.

Foods to Avoid

The average North American diet is full of heavily processed foods, including packaged foods and fast food. These items tend to have unhealthy amounts of sodium and sugar. They also often contain trans fat, which is highly inflammatory and can lead to heart disease.

The best way to buy groceries is to focus on the things that are located on the perimeter of the supermarket. That's where you will find fresh produce, fresh meat and fish, and dairy products. The interior aisles are where you will find packaged foods, frozen foods, and many of the things that are the least healthy to eat. It may not be possible to avoid the interior aisles completely, but if the majority of your food comes from the perimeter you will be eliminating many cancer-causing ingredients from your diet.
It is important to note that some things in the interior aisles, such as plain frozen vegetables, are perfectly acceptable. However, it is still best to look for organic options.

Foods that Help Prevent Cancer

I would like to close the chapter by highlighting a few foods that have known cancer-fighting properties.

- Cruciferous vegetables such as broccoli, cauliflower, cabbage, and kale are powerful allies in the fight against cancer. Broccoli is especially effective since it contains sulforaphane, which helps to flush cancer-causing chemicals out of the body.

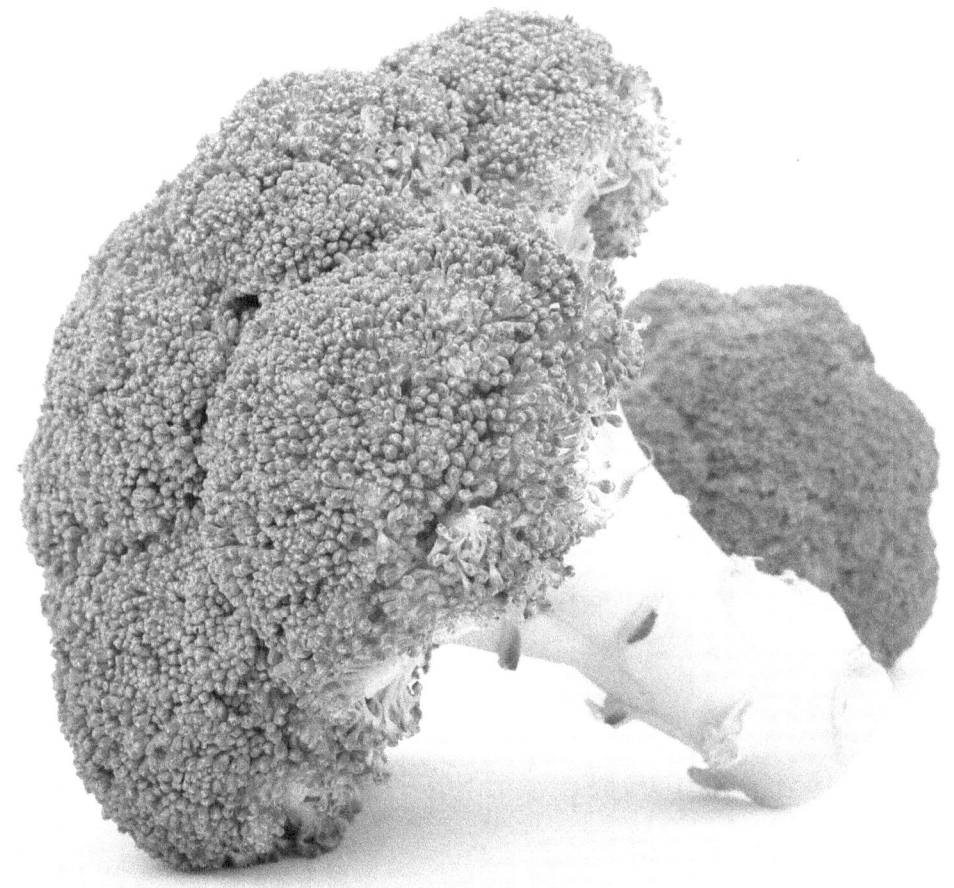

- Berries are a rich source of antioxidants known as anthocyanins, which can slow the growth of cancer cells and prevent the formation of new blood vessels that might feed tumors.
- Tomatoes contain lycopene, a carotenoid that is responsible for their bright red color. It has been shown to help prevent several kinds of cancer, including endometrial cancer, prostate cancer, lung cancer, and stomach cancer.
- Walnuts are a rich source of phytosterols, which have been shown to block the estrogen receptors in breast cancer cells. They may also help to prevent prostate cancer.
- Garlic contains phytochemicals that may slow or halt the body's absorption of harmful nitrates, which can lead to gastrointestinal cancer.
- Red grapes are a good source of resveratrol, a chemical that may help to slow the growth of cancer cells.
- Turmeric is a spice that is widely used in Indian cooking. It is also one of the world's most powerful antioxidants and may help to prevent age-related cancers.
- Whole grains are preferable to foods made with refined flour thanks to their fiber content. Fiber helps flush out the colon and may help to prevent colon cancer.

Other foods that are beneficial include green tea, dark chocolate, apples, beans, and dark leafy greens like spinach.

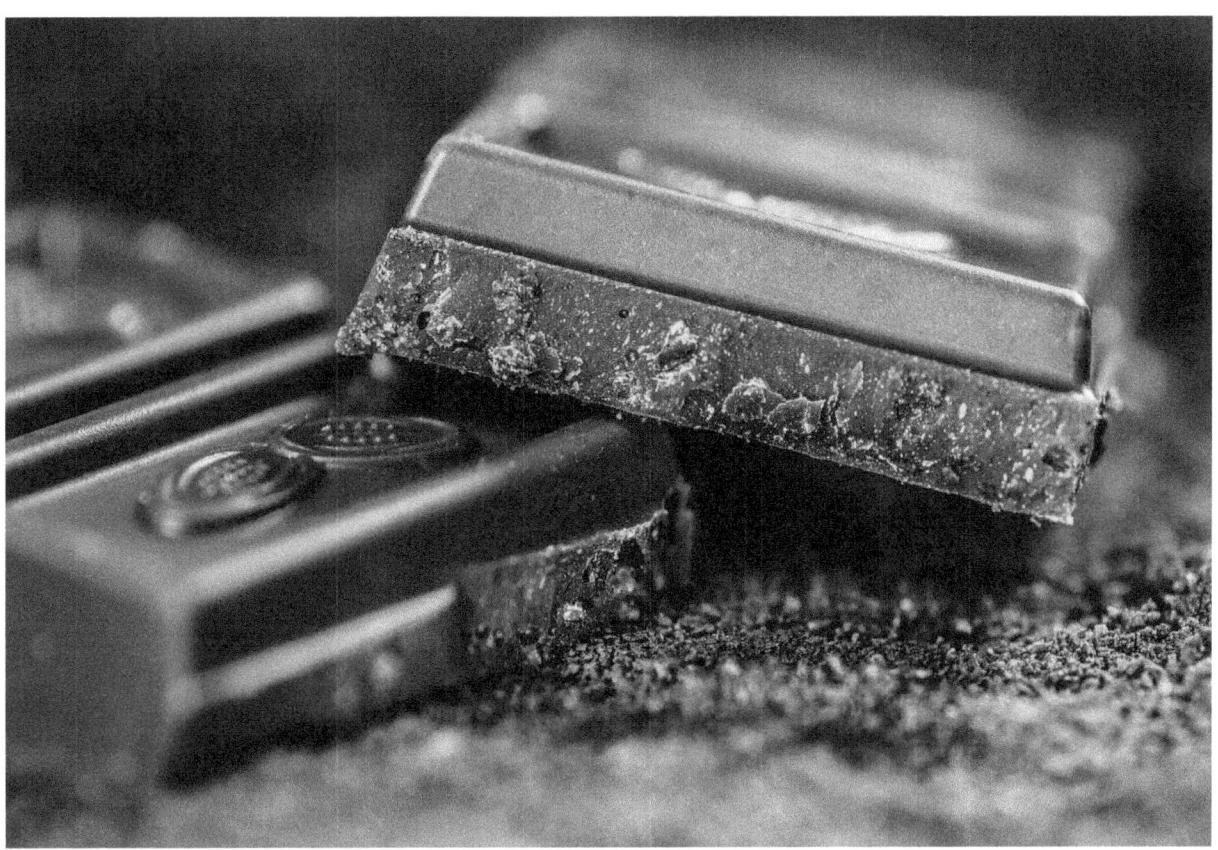

If the majority of your diet is plant-based and organic, you will be giving your body much of what it needs to keep you cancer-free and healthy. In the next chapter, we'll talk about vitamins and supplements and how they can help prevent cancer. ****If You Enjoy the Info So Far Click Here to Join Our Email List****

Anti-Cancer Vitamins

Nutritional supplements are one of the most popular forms of natural healing. Many of us take a host of supplements every day. We turn to supplements to help us fight chronic ailments and avoid the use of prescription drugs. It should come as no surprise that there are some supplements that can help prevent cancer.

The Dangers of Vitamin Deficiencies

In the last chapter, I talked about the role that Vitamin C plays in your body. Micronutrients get their name because we require very small amounts of them to be healthy – in some cases, only a few milligrams per day. However, those small amounts are essential and if we don't get them, we can do serious damage to our health.

Let's use Vitamin C as an example again. In the past, when access to fresh produce was limited, many people ended up with a condition called scurvy, the result of a Vitamin C deficiency. A vitamin deficiency is defined as a condition in which a person is chronically deprived of an essential micronutrient. Scurvy can cause weakness, fatigue, slow wound healing, bleeding gums, and bruising.

Other vitamin deficiencies can be equally as dangerous. Vitamin D deficiency is fairly common, especially in geographical areas that don't get much sunlight. As much as 32% of the United States population is estimated to be Vitamin D deficient. Some of the symptoms of deficiency include skeletal weakness, aching joints, depression, and headaches.

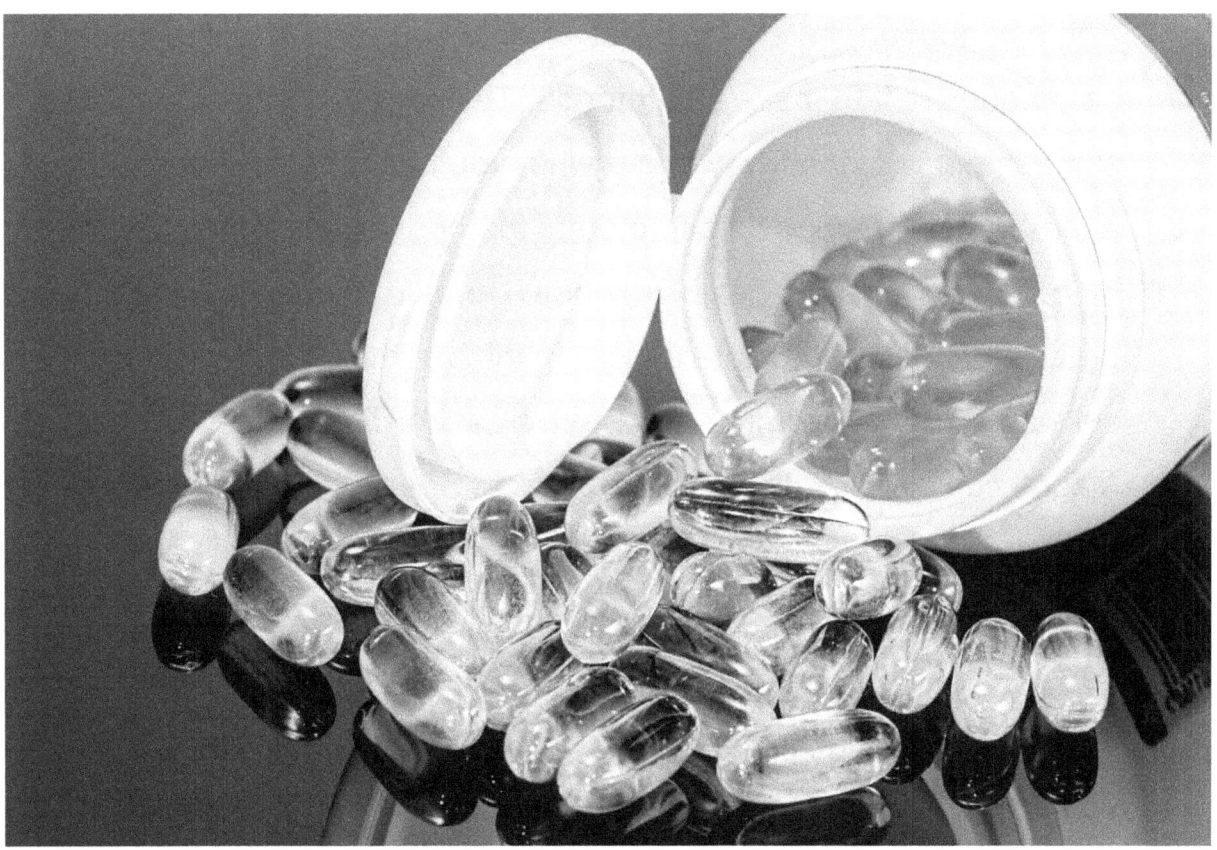

Supplements to Take to Prevent Cancer

Nutritionists will tell you that it is best to get the vitamins and minerals you need from food, and for the most part, that's true. However, in some cases it may be a real challenge to get enough of a particular nutrient from your diet. Here are some of the supplements I recommend to my patients.

- Vitamin D, deficiency, as I said before, is relatively common. Inadequate Vitamin D intake has been linked to breast cancer. If you live in an area that doesn't get much sun or you have dark skin, you may want to consider taking a Vitamin D supplement.
- You can add turmeric to your diet, but many people find it difficult to get enough of it to make a difference. Taking a turmeric or curcumin supplement is a good way to get what you need. Its powerful antioxidant properties help to protect the body from cancer.
- Zinc supplementation has been shown to help people who have breast cancer and prostate cancer. It inhibits the growth of cancer cells and boosts the immune system's cancer-fighting power.
- Magnesium is essential for maintaining a healthy digestive system. One study showed that for every additional 100 milligrams of magnesium patients took, their risk of colon cancer declined by about 13%.
- Omega-3 essential fatty acid is an important part of any diet, but if you don't eat fish you may not be getting enough of it. There is research to suggest that the best kind of Omega-3 to take comes from krill oil, a renewable resource that is not subject to mercury contamination. However, vegetarians and vegans can get what they need from flaxseed oil.
- Probiotics can help maintain the health of your digestive system and promote the growth of healthy bacteria. These bacteria can neutralize carcinogenic substances.

- Ellagic acid is a substance found in many berries. It promotes a process known as apoptosis – the killing of abnormal cells that can lead to cancer.

If you eat a diet rich in fruits, vegetables, whole grains, and lean proteins, and take these supplements, you can be sure that your body has what it needs to fight cancer.

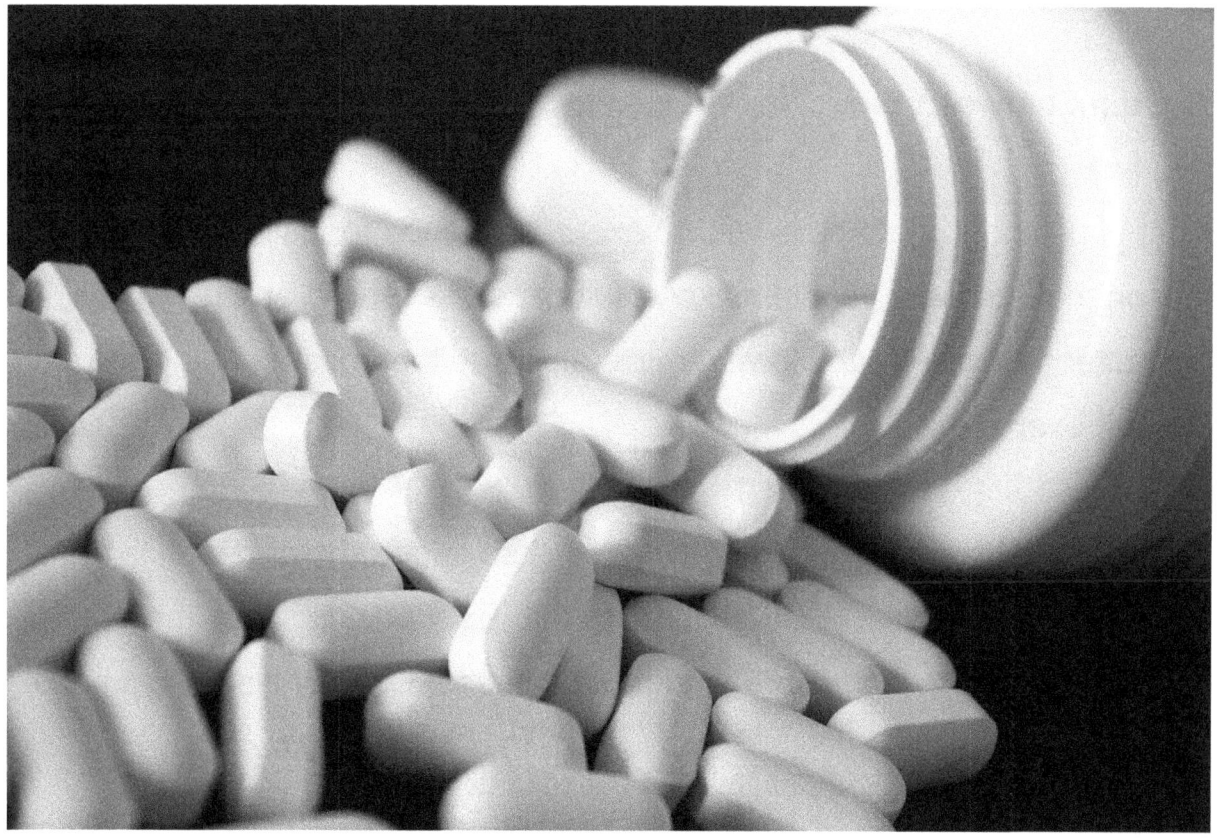

Of course, diet alone is not enough to prevent cancer. The next chapter will look at the cancer-fighting benefits of exercise.

Anti-Cancer Exercise

In the not-too-distant past, the majority of people spent their days engaged in physical activity of one kind or another. Their jobs were active, whether they were working in a factory, on a farm, or inside the home. Today, however, many of the manual jobs that we did ourselves in the past have been taken over by machines. As a result, our physical fitness has decreased and cancer rates have increased.

The Link between Exercise and Health

Most of us know on some level that exercise is good for us. There's a reason that so many people make resolutions to exercise and join gyms right after the New Year. However, it is also true that most of us do not get enough exercise.

One of the primary reasons that exercise is so important for health is that it helps prevent obesity, which is linked to many serious diseases including diabetes, high blood pressure, and heart disease. Obesity also plays a role in certain cancers, especially colon cancer and other cancers of the digestive tract.

The human body is meant to move. If we want our hearts and lungs to be healthy, we have to make them work. Sitting behind a desk all day does very little to promote cardiovascular health or prevent obesity.

How Exercise Helps Prevent Cancer

How does exercise help prevent cancer? Let's look at some of the concrete benefits that come from exercising regularly.

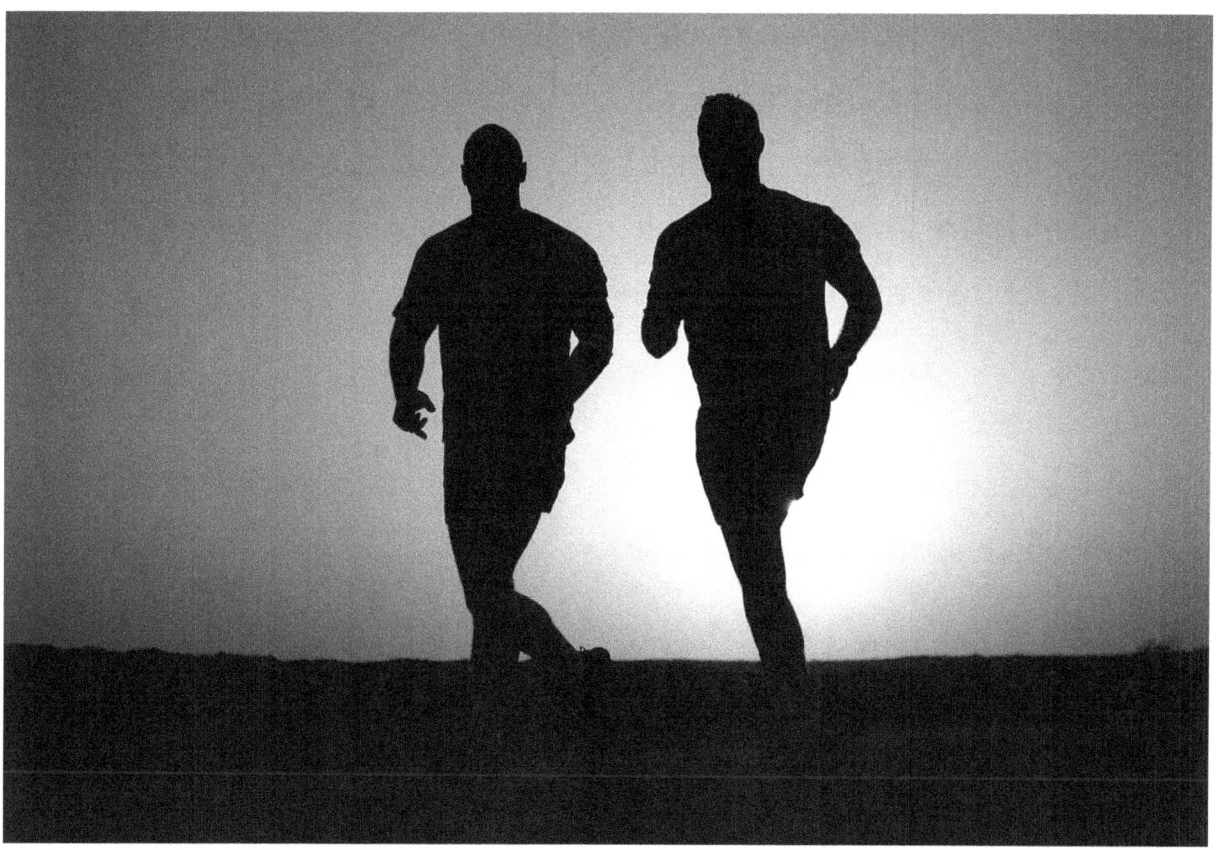

1. Women who exercise regularly have a 30% to 40% lower risk of breast cancer than those who do not exercise. The reason is that breast cancer is linked to estrogen levels in the blood and regular exercise helps to keep estrogen in check. This is especially important for women who are post-menopausal, since after menopause estrogen is produced by fat cells. Weight gain becomes more likely as we age.

2. Exercise helps to regulate insulin levels in the body, and insulin is another risk factor for cancer. Having excess insulin may lead to other health problems as well, including insulin resistance, weight gain, and diabetes.
3. Regular exercise changes the chemical composition of the digestive system and, as a result, protects against colorectal cancer. More than 250,000 people are diagnosed with colon cancer every year, and obesity is a contributing factor as well. One thing that is affected by exercise are levels of growth hormones, which can contribute to the development and growth of cancer cells.

As you can see, exercise is very important in cancer prevention. Regular exercise, especially when it is combined with an anti-cancer diet and proper nutrition, can help decrease your risk.

Anti-Cancer Exercise Guidelines and Tips

When I talk to my patients about exercise, I generally recommend that they get a minimum of 30 minutes of exercise every day. The more vigorous the exercise, the more dramatic the health benefits. However, for patients who are sedentary and unaccustomed to exercise, my initial suggestion is that they go for a brisk walk every day. Walking is incredibly beneficial and relatively easy for people to incorporate into their daily routine.

Here are some other suggestions to help you get the anti-cancer benefits of exercise:

- Pick a form of exercise that you like, as you are more likely to stick with it than you would be if you picked something you hate. Not a fan of jogging? Try swimming laps at the pool instead.

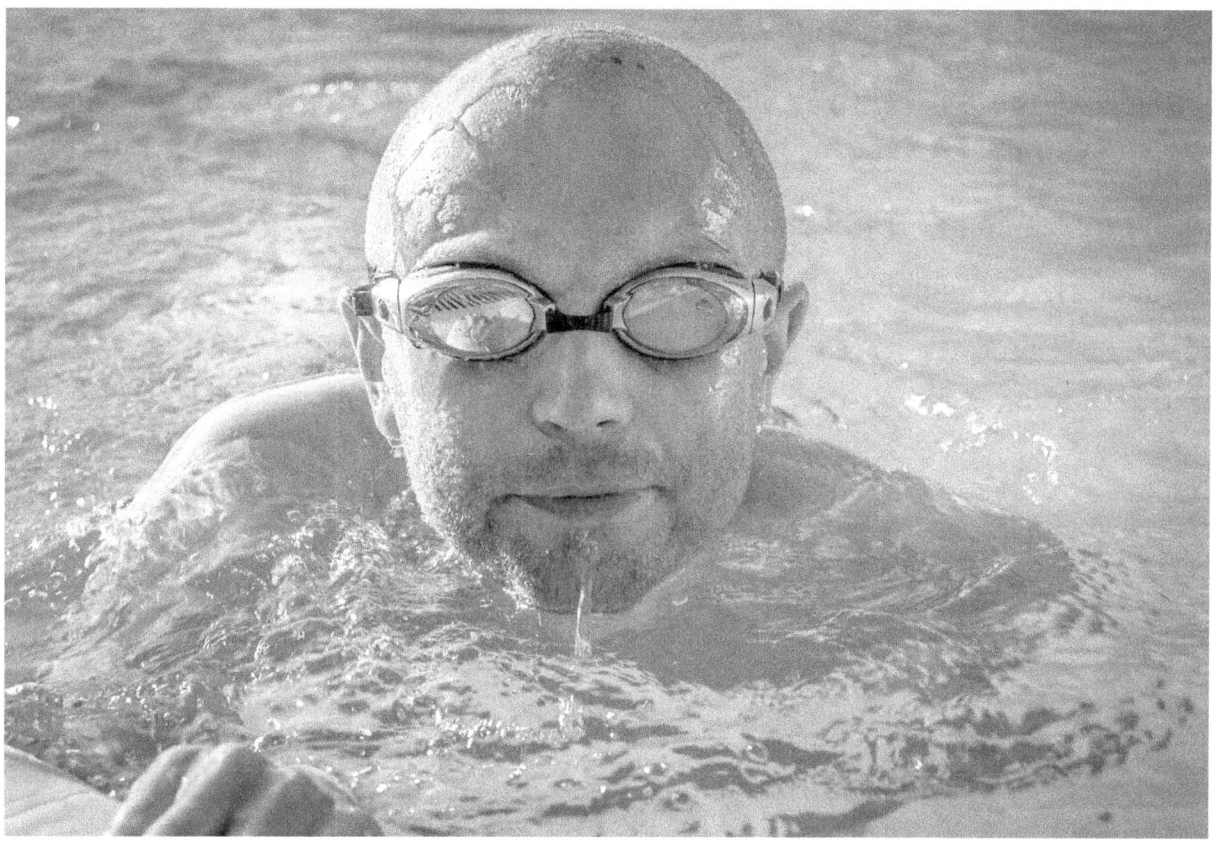

- Exercise with a buddy. We may find excuses to skip exercising if we do it alone, but having a partner makes it easy to hold ourselves accountable.
- Find opportunities to increase physical activity. Examples including walking short distances instead of driving, taking the stairs at work, and playing with your kids instead of sitting in front of the television.

- If the idea of exercise doesn't appeal to you, try something really basic like buying a pedometer and keeping track of your steps. Many people who claim not to like exercise get caught up in trying to increase the number of steps they take each day.

Exercise helps control your weight, regulate hormones, and keep your digestive system healthy.

In the next chapter, I will talk about a particular type of exercise that I feel is particularly beneficial for cancer prevention: Yoga.

Anti-Cancer Yoga

Yoga is a form of exercise that has been practiced for centuries. It has reached new popularity in the United States in recent years, with many gyms offering hot yoga classes and touting the benefits of doing Yoga.

Yoga is good exercise, and it is also one of the most effective things you can do to help prevent cancer.

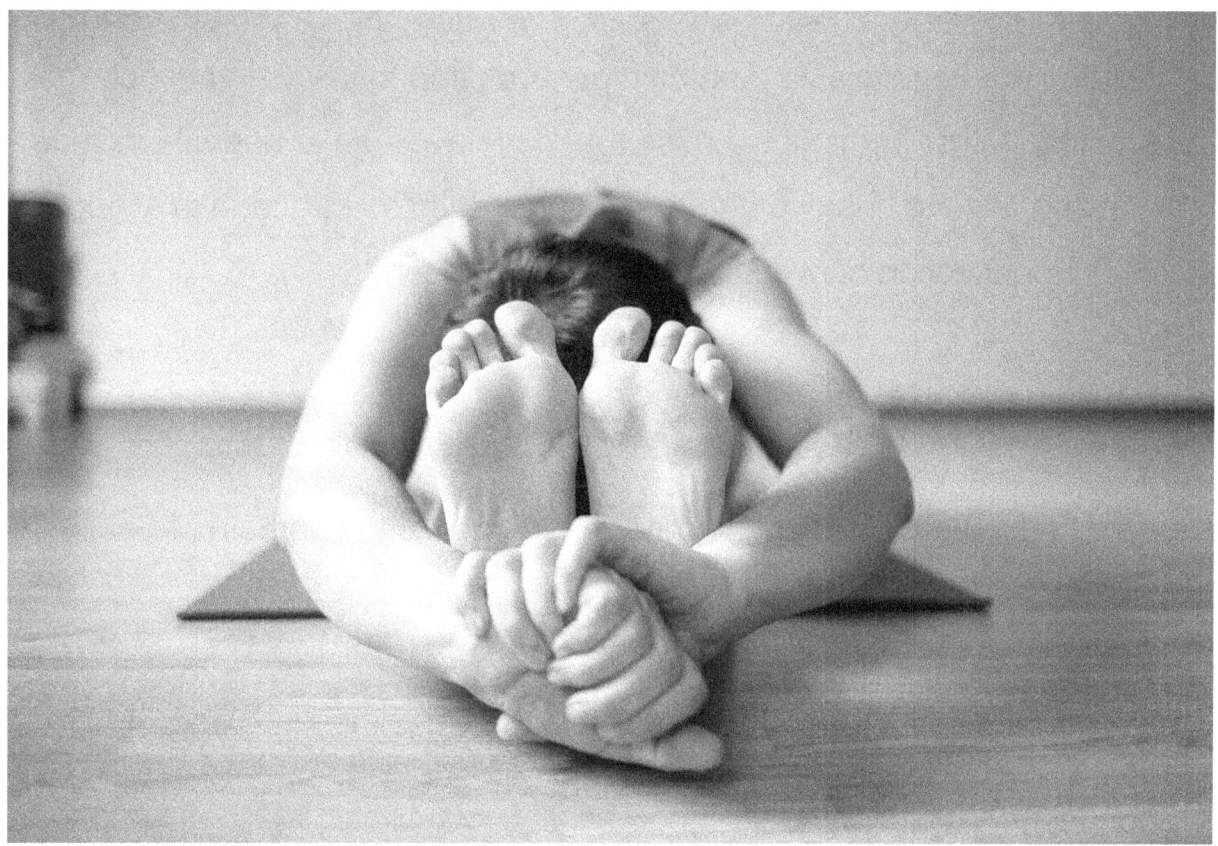

How Strengthening the Mind-Body Connection Prevents Cancer

I want to start by talking about the connection between the mind and the body. People who have a positive mindset tend to be physically and mentally healthier than those who do not. Research shows that things like negativity, anxiety, and stress can be detrimental to physical health. Stress, for example, is directly linked to things like depression, high blood pressure, heart disease, digestive problems, and more.

Forms of exercise that help reduce stress and strengthen the mind-body connection are beneficial for health in general, and for reducing cancer risk in particular. Other forms of exercise that can have similar benefits include T'ai chi and qi gong. Many of the martial arts, such as karate, also work on building a connection between the body and the mind.

Health Benefits of Yoga

Now let's talk about the specific ways that doing Yoga can help protect you from cancer.

1. Yoga strengthens the lymphatic system, which helps to detoxify the body. The specific breathing and movements of yoga activate the lymphatic system. Inverted postures are particularly helpful for reversing the effects of gravity and increasing lymphatic and cardiovascular drainage. Moves that incorporate twists also help detoxify the body by briefly compressing internal organs.

2. Yoga strengthens the immune system, which helps the body fight diseases and infections. People who have strong immunity are better able to resist cancer than those who don't. A 2013 Norwegian study found that Yoga practice helped increase circulation of cancer-fighting cells.

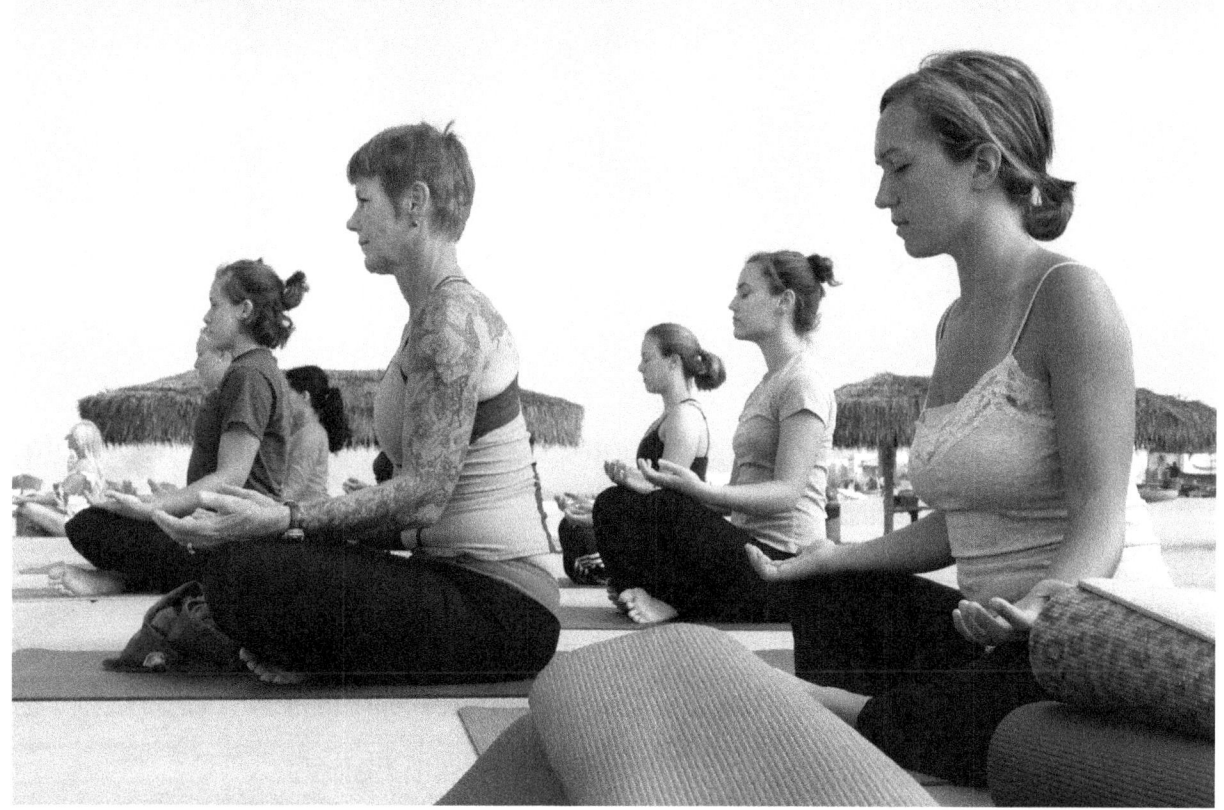

3. Yoga builds strong bones, thus increasing leukocyte (white blood cell) production in the bones. Leukocytes are an important part of your body's cancer-fighting arsenal.
4. Yoga helps with weight management. We have already talked about the link between obesity and cancer. While intense cardiovascular

exercise is important, active Yoga where practitioners are constantly in motion burns calories and revs up the metabolism.
5. Yoga reduces stress. Various studies have shown that cancer increases positive feelings and decreases stress and anxiety.

As you can see, the practice of Yoga is one that can do quite a lot to keep your body free of cancer.

Tips for Doing Yoga

Here are some tips to help you incorporate the practice of Yoga into your life:

- Practice active Yoga that concentrates on the flow of movement from position to position.
- Yoga is most effective when it is part of a workout routine that also includes intense aerobic activity and weight training.
- Practicing Yoga three times a week for thirty minutes is a good way to form a healthy habit and reap all of the health benefits.
- If you have never practiced Yoga before, you may want to seek out a class locally or look for an online class to ensure that you are doing it properly.
- Begin with relatively easy poses and work your way up to more challenging poses. People who practice Yoga for years can often do arm stands and other advanced poses. Have realistic expectations

and start slowly. It is better to do that than to injure yourself by attempting something that your body is unprepared to do.

Yoga is great exercise and a powerful way to prevent cancer. In the next chapter, we will talk about some of the products we put into our bodies and how they can impact our risk of getting cancer.

Anti-Cancer Products

How aware are you of the products you put into and on your body? When you scan a list of ingredients, do you know what they are? If you are using all-natural soap made with goat milk and olive oil, this chapter might not apply to you. However, if your bathroom and kitchen are full of products that contain chemicals with unpronounceable names, then it is essential for you to be more mindful of what you put into your body.

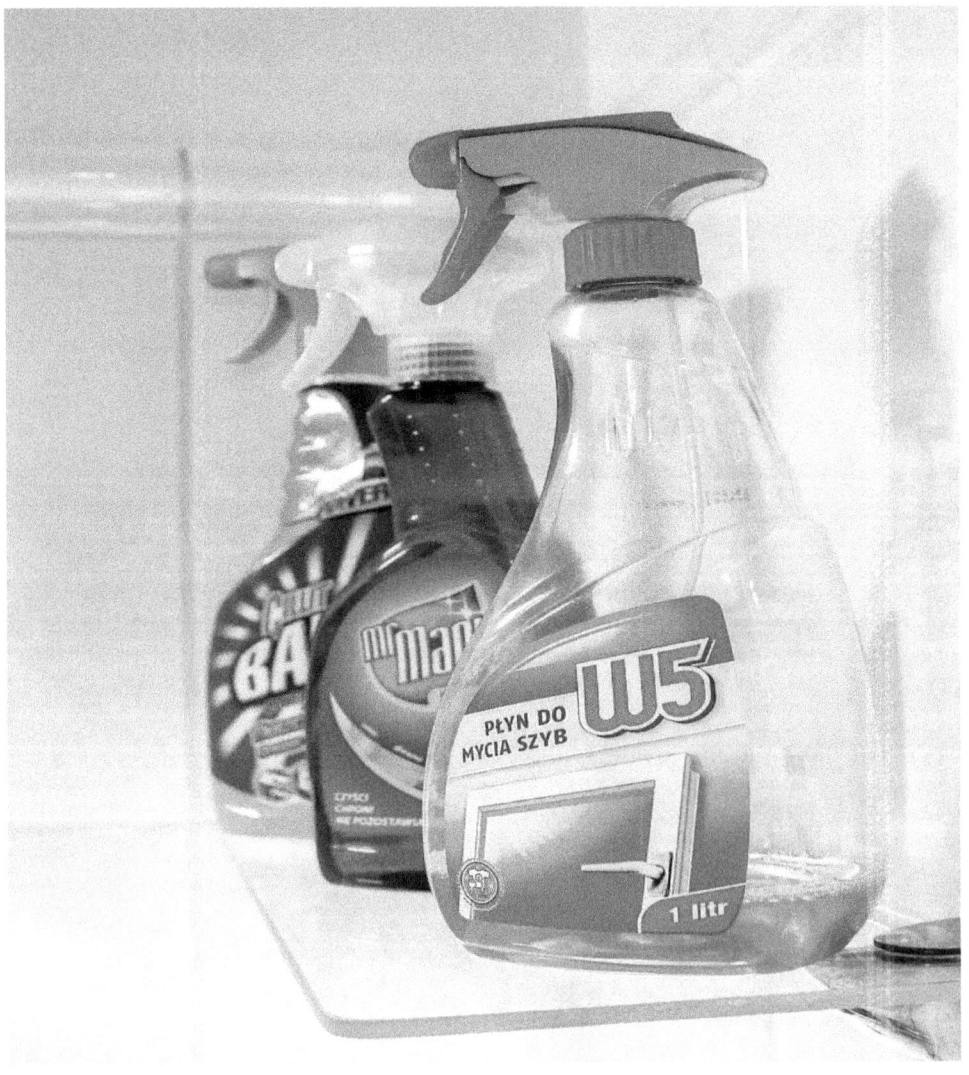

The Link between Chemicals and Cancer

The conversation about toxic chemicals and cancer has been happening for a long time. Rachel Carson's landmark book, <u>Silent Spring</u>, looked at the effect that chemicals were having on the environment. Today, there is increasing concern that we are routinely exposing ourselves to carcinogenic substances in our makeup and beauty products, and in cleaning products too.

Some chemicals and products are so toxic that we have already banned them – think of the effort to get rid of asbestos as an example. However, the fact remains that many of us use chemicals every day that can cause or contribute to cancer. Some of the chemicals that are most associated with cancer include benzene, arsenic, formaldehyde, and isopropyl alcohol. One chemical that is being scrutinized in 2016 is cocamide DEA, which is an ingredient in many popular brands of shampoo. It is important to know what the ingredients in your favorite products are.

Chemicals to Avoid

What I recommend to my patients is that they pull out all of their cosmetics, beauty products, and cleaning products and take an inventory of ingredients. Here are the most common ingredients that you should avoid:

- Urea
- Parabens

- Phthalates
- Propylene glycol and polyethylene glycol
- Petroleum by-products
- Sodium laurel sulfate and sodium laureth sulfate
- Diethanolamine (DEA) and triethanolamine (TEA)
- Formaldehyde
- Benzene
- Cocamide DEA
- EDTA and disodium EDTA
- Toluene
- Triclosan
- Silicone-derived emollients
- Hydroquinone

Of course, this is only a partial list. If you are unsure about an ingredient, I strongly encourage you to look it up and decide if it is something you want to use.

Replacements for Unhealthy Products

After you remove harmful products from your home, you need some information about what to use instead. Here are some suggestions:

- In many cases, all-natural products such as lemon juice, salt, vinegar, and baking soda make excellent cleaning products.

- Castile soap is a very gentle, natural soap that can be used in a variety of ways.
- Soaps made with natural ingredients like olive oil, almond oil, goat milk, and essential oils will get you just as clean as commercial products without the health risks.
- The same goes for all-natural shampoos and conditioners. They may not foam the way some products do, but keep in mind that the foam is often caused by the very chemicals you are trying to avoid.
- Instead of using moisturizers that are laden with chemicals, try using a gentle, all-natural moisturizer like extra virgin coconut oil. You can use it on your face and body, and you can buy a jar that will last you for months for less than ten dollars.

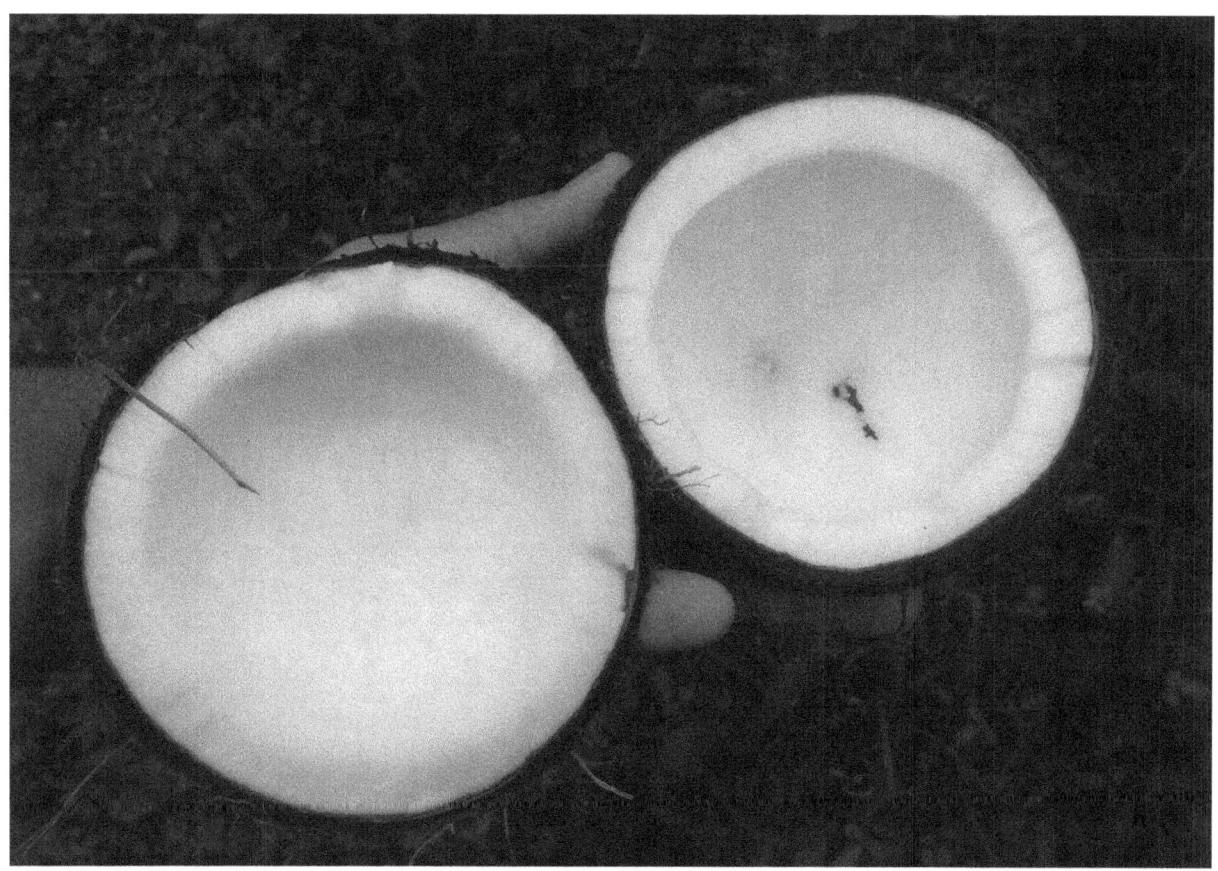

If you do a bit of research, you can find all-natural products (or make them yourself) that will work just as well as the products that are full of dangerous chemicals.

Now that we've covered diet, exercise, and chemicals, it's time to tackle our last topic: creating habits that help to fight cancer.

Anti-Cancer Habits

In this last chapter, I want to talk about a variety of things that you probably do (or don't do) in your everyday life that may be contributing to your risk of getting cancer. It is sometimes said that it takes only 21 days to build a new habit. When I talk to my patients about cancer prevention, I always encourage them to start making small changes immediately. Many of these things may require you to be mindful at first, but if you stick to them, they will quickly become habits.

The Habits that Prevent Cancer

While the things we have already discussed – nutrition, supplementation, exercise, Yoga, and chemicals – can all help you reduce your risk of getting cancer, there is still more that you can do. Here are some of the healthy habits I suggest you adopt.

1. Filter the water you use for drinking and cooking. The lead contamination in Flint, Michigan shone a spotlight on the problem with municipal water supplies. The best way to protect your family is to invest in water filters for your home. Effective filters will eliminate much of the chemical content and environmental toxins in your water, making it safe to drink.
2. Make sure to get enough sleep. Sleep is essential for human health. When you sleep, your body rids itself of biochemical waste. Sleep also helps to reduce stress and anxiety. The average adult needs

between seven and nine hours of sleep per night. Children need more. A good way to tell how much sleep you need is to track how long you sleep on days when you don't need an alarm to get up. Then set a sleep schedule that allow you to go to bed and get up at the same time every day.

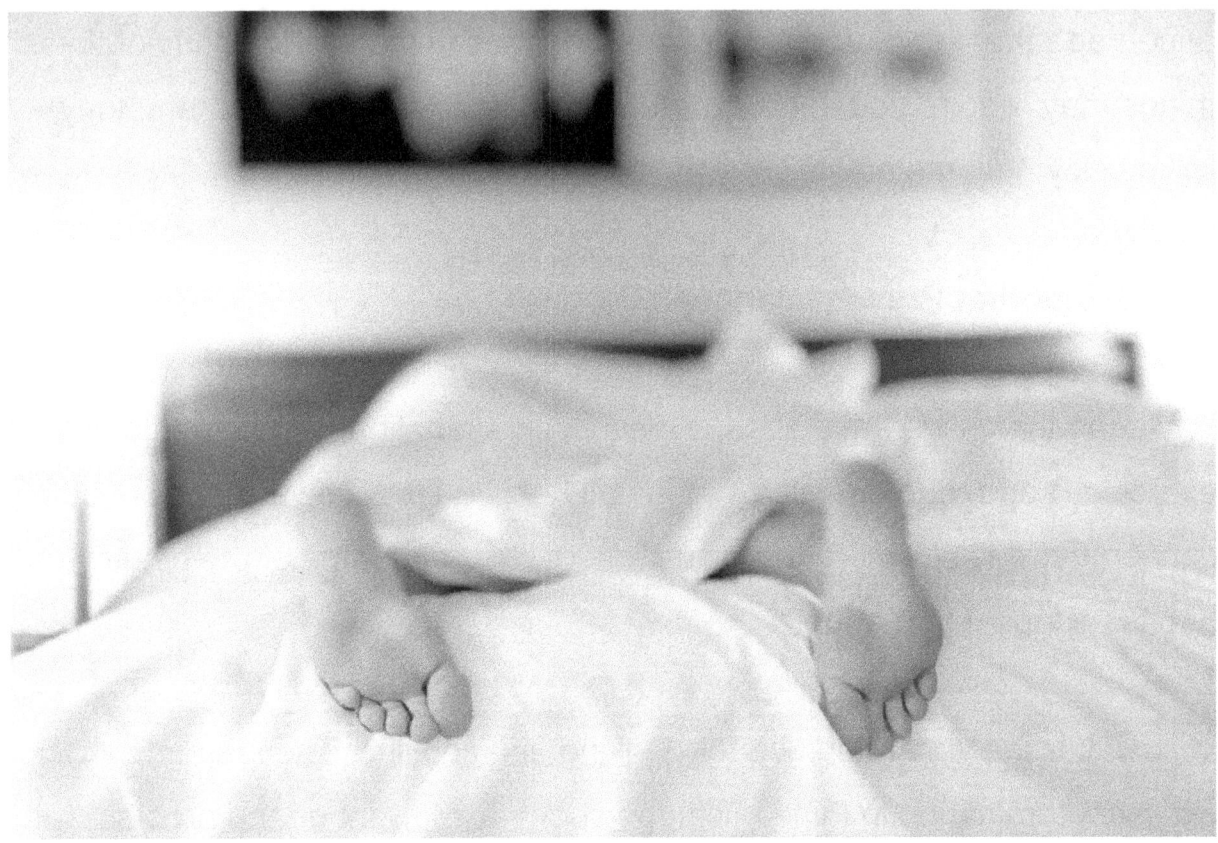

3. Always wear sunscreen. While we all need Vitamin D, many of us thoughtlessly expose ourselves to unhealthy levels of radiation every day. In fact, most of us put on sunscreen only when we will be spending a day at the beach or the pool. If your skin is exposed to the sun – which it is even on cloudy days – you should be wearing sunscreen. Make sure to choose a natural sunscreen that is free of

dangerous chemicals. You and your children should wear it every day to reduce your risk of getting skin cancer.

4. Find ways to reduce your levels of stress. We talked a bit about stress in the chapter about Yoga, but it is important to talk about some of the other things you can do to minimize stress. Many of us spend our days in a state of perpetual stress. It can wreak havoc with our bodies, keeping us in a perpetual state of "fight or flight." We have unhealthy levels of stress hormones, including adrenaline and cortisol. These can cause us to gain weight, and contribute to things like high blood pressure, heart disease, and depression. Some of the things that may help to reduce stress are meditation, exercise, play, creativity, and having a support system of people to whom you can turn when you are overwhelmed.

5. Don't use any kind of tobacco product. Smoking is not as popular as it once was, but many people use e-cigs or vape as a substitute. Many of the same chemicals are included in these products that are in regular cigarettes, and they can do serious damage to your body.

6. Limit your intake of alcoholic beverages. Moderate alcohol intake is acceptable and may even be healthy. For example, research suggests that drinking limited amounts of red wine may improve cardiac health. However, heavy drinking can damage your liver, which is one of your body's primary detoxification organs. Try to limit your intake to one or (at most) two drinks per day.

7. Avoid risky behavior such as unprotected sex or needle sharing. Human papillomavirus is one of the most common sexually transmitted diseases, and it is a known precursor to cervical cancer.

Use condoms unless you are in a long-term committed relationship and have both been tested. Never share needles at any time.

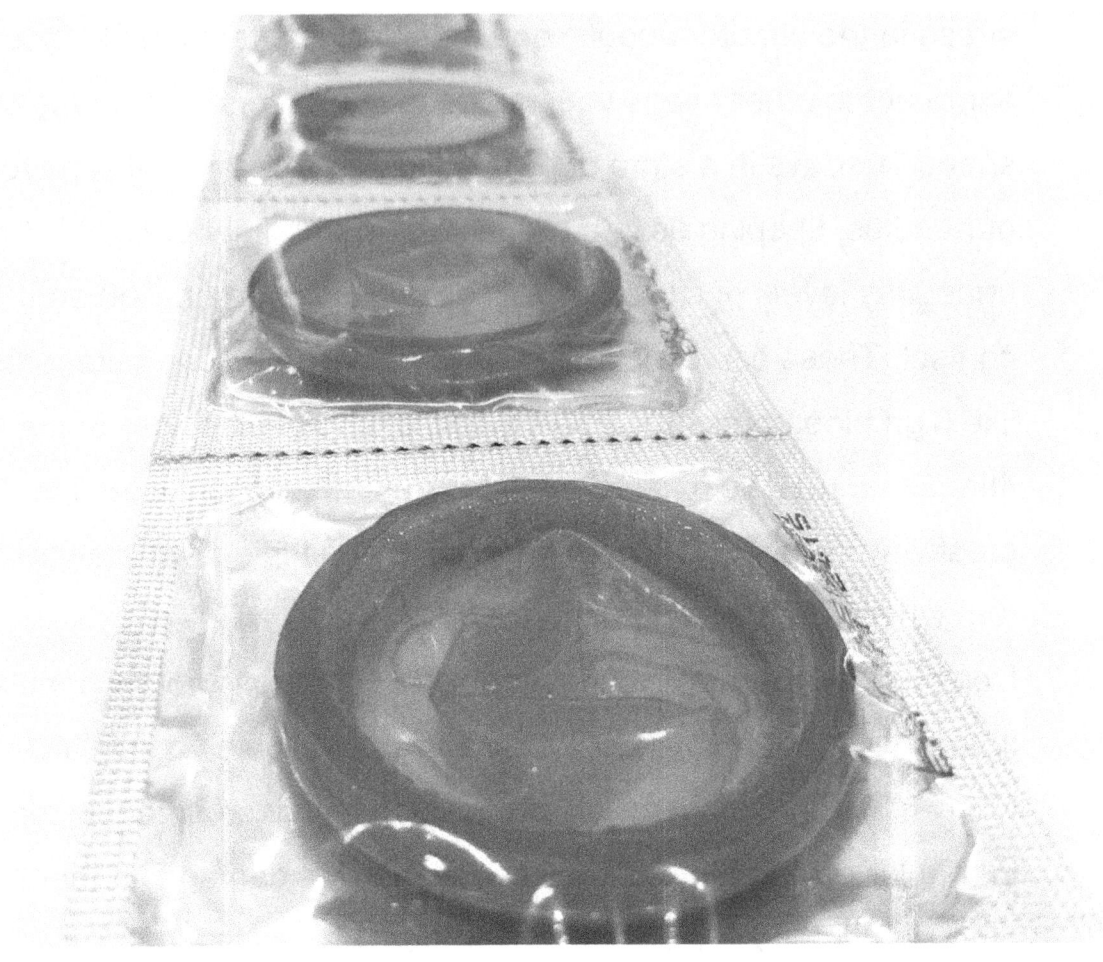

8. Get regular check-ups and cancer screenings. Women should have regular mammograms and PAP smears, and do monthly breast exams at home. All men should get regular prostate exams. People of both sexes need colonoscopies to check for colon cancer, and get regular skin cancer screenings, too.

These eight habits can do a great deal to reduce your chances of getting cancer. Regular screenings will ensure that even if you do get cancer, it will be caught early when treatments are likely to be effective and survival rates are high.

A few simple changes can help protect you and your family from cancer.

Conclusion

Thank you for reading *Taboo Cancer Cures*. It is not possible to completely eliminate the possibility that you will get cancer, but if you follow the simple and practical steps outlined in this book, you can be confident that you are doing what you can to minimize your risk.

As a quick recap, here are the things you can do starting today to keep yourself and your family healthy:

- Eat a healthy diet of whole, natural foods and avoid processed foods
- Take nutritional supplements as needed, including Vitamin D, magnesium, zinc, curcumin, probiotics, ellagic acid, and Omega-3.
- Get at least 30 minutes of aerobic exercise most days. The American Cancer Society recommends a total of 150 minutes per week.
- Take up Yoga as a way of strengthening the mind-body connection, detoxifying your body, and burning fat.
- Scan your household for products that contain harmful chemicals and replace them with natural, non-carcinogenic products.
- Build healthy habits: filter your water, get enough sleep, reduce stress, wear sunscreen, don't use tobacco, limit alcohol consumption, avoid risky behavior, and get regular cancer screenings.

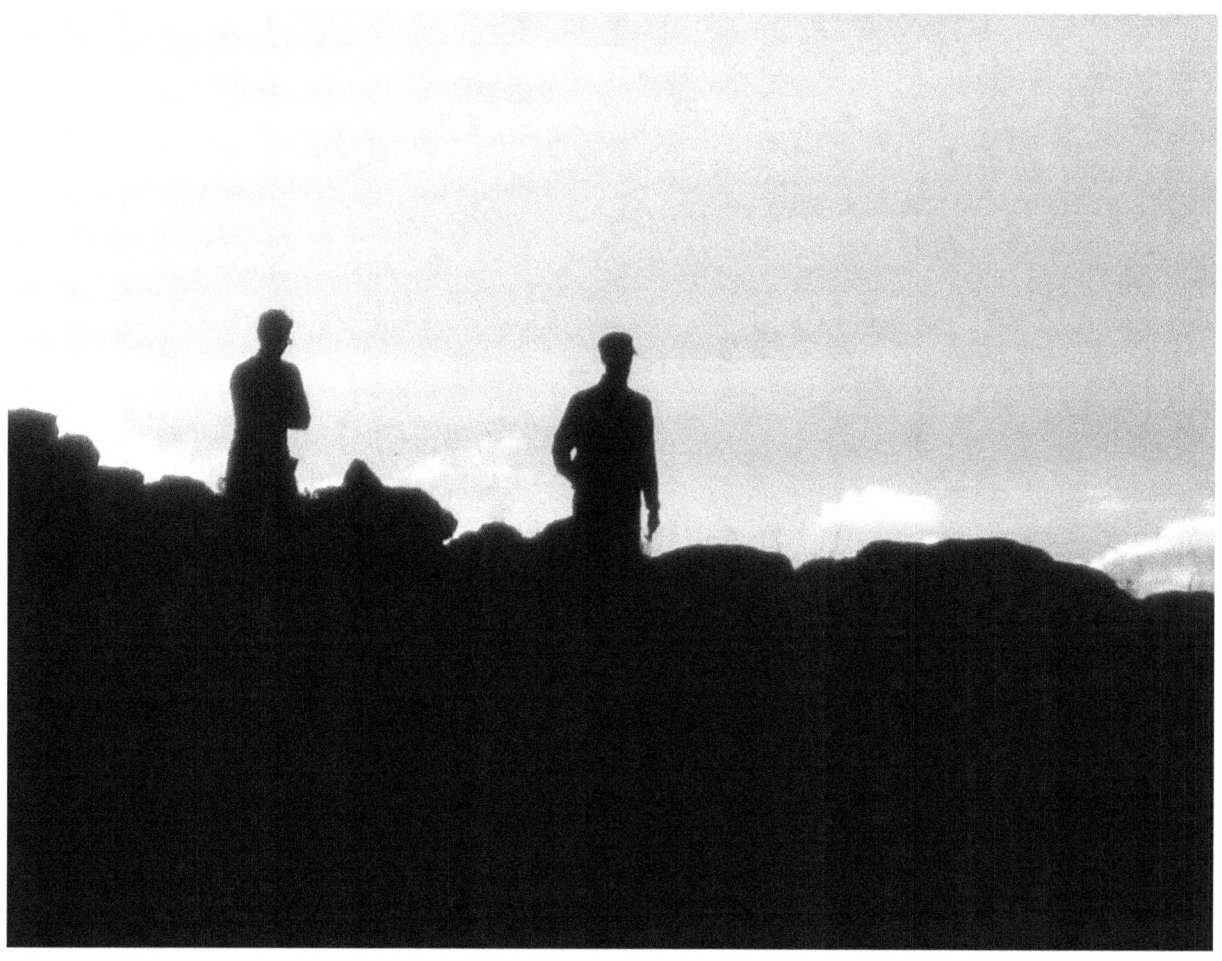

If you do these things, your body will have what it needs to fight cancer and keep you strong and healthy for years to come.

www.ingramcontent.com/pod-product-compliance
Lightning Source LLC
Chambersburg PA
CBHW080525190526
45169CB00008B/3059